Dedicated to my father who taught me to love and respect horses.

Hadley Incorporated

Cover Design:
Holly Nichols

Editors:
Julia Nichols
Kate Capra
Jennifer Ramsey

Publication disclaimer:

www. equinehusbands.com

Table of Contents

Preface

Having been in equine practice for the last 14 years I have had numerous experiences that led me to write this book. Most of my clients are women. Why this is I am not sure, but they often seem to have a special bond with horses and often grow much more attached to them. If you are married to, dating, or trying to date one of these women it behooves you to have some clue about horses and their health issues. This will not only make you appear less ignorant when socializing with "horse people," but it will also give you an idea of what to do when your significant other is gone and you are charged with caring for the steed. This knowledge may help prevent divorce, breakup, or worse if a horse gets sick or injured on your watch. In this book you will find some basic information to help maintain your happy home.

Lets start in with some "up front" information that will help you if your wife is just getting started in horses or had one as a child and now is continuing to fulfill her life long dream of horse ownership.

Now prepare for the worst. Horse ownership has been compared to standing over a toilet, opening your wallet and flushing all the money down the drain. Horses are very expensive to maintain besides the fact that it will be your wife's goal to accessorize herself and the horse.

The cost of buying the horse is only a drop in the bucket so you might as well get a good one to start with. There is hay, grain, shelter (or boarding fees), horse shoers, and last, but not least, veterinary costs. Then show fees, a horse trailer, a bigger vehicle to pull it with that will use more gas. Next comes a new saddle or two, depending on the particular occasion. Then tack for the horse and proper riding attire for your wife. I am sure that an experienced horse husband could add to this list.

Eventually your wife will discover the huge numbers of horse paraphernalia catalogs that are in circulation. She will become convinced that there are many more items that she can't live without such as liniments, bandages, and an endless supply of feed supplements. I would suggest that she consult with her vet before purchasing too many of these items. I have actually seen horses ruined by over-feeding these additives, so help her to be a wary consumer. Remember to tread lightly when making suggestions. Your rank in the family has already dropped since the horse came on the scene, so don't make it worse for yourself.

Now that you have heard the bad news, let me tell you the good news. The horse will keep your wife occupied for hours on end. This will give you time to watch football on T.V. and hang with the boys. You will also form a whole new circle of friends, other horse husbands. An important group that you can commiserate with. Your wife will also expect you to join her at some equine social events and as long as you can talk the talk you should be able to get through it.

I hope that by reading this book you will be better prepared for your role as "horse husband." Good luck and may the strong survive.

USED HORSES

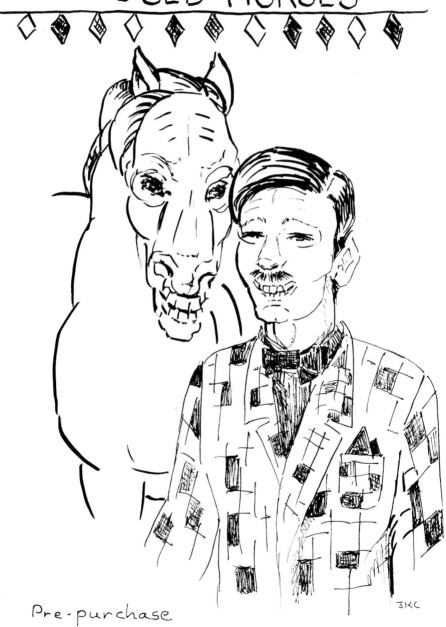

Pre-purchase

The Pre-Purchase Exam

"But Doc, they told me that he wasn't more than five years old and had never taken a lame step."

When buying a new horse, it is most important not to get ripped off unnecessarily. Purchasing a new horse is similar to buying a used car. You are never told exactly what you are getting and often shady characters are involved. When you start looking at a particular horse, it is a good idea to find out as much about the seller as possible. This information can usually be obtained from other "horse people" in the community. You will quickly find out who you want to deal with and who you don't. Purchasing a horse is a "buyer beware" situation. Once you have laid down the cash, there is rarely a good return policy. My recommendation is that no matter who you are buying the horse from, neighbor, relative, or friend, you should always have a veterinarian perform a pre-purchase exam, or, shall we say, "have a look under the hood."

It is considered poor form to have the seller's veterinarian do this exam. Pick your own veterinarian, preferably one who has not seen the animal before. One word of advice, "man to man," – have this exam done before your wife falls in love with the horse, just in case a major problem is discovered and the horse is deemed unfit. I can cite numerous situations when I've found a major health problem on a pre-purchase exam, but the wife has already fallen in love with the horse. The unknowing husband is then stuck buying a disabled horse that will probably cost a fortune in veterinary services or special shoeing over the next several years.

Another common mistake is to buy the horse first, then call a veterinarian for a post-purchase exam. This is often a waste of time, because if a major problem is found at this point, it is probably too late to return the horse. Additionally, your wife may make you sleep in the barn should you even suggest returning the animal. Now that the seller is counting your money, what you may have is an expensive lawn ornament. Meanwhile, your wife is looking for another horse that she can actually ride!

The pre-purchase exam involves a thorough examination of the horse from head to tail. I tell my clients upfront that the "perfect horse" does not exist. All horses have some sort of flaw.

A common and very disappointing finding is that the seller has misrepresented the animal's age. When I must tell the "ready to ride buyer" that the horse is actually 20 years older than they were told, they are quite disappointed. Age can be determined by using the front teeth as a gauge. When the seller hears that there is an age discrepancy, he or she usually stomps around determined to find some official papers to prove the veterinarian wrong. At this point, you should walk away.

Other problems often found in a pre-purchase exam range from past surgeries and medical procedures, to chronic lameness or respiratory damage, but the aspect of the exam that often gets the most attention is the feet and legs. There is an old horseman's saying that should be taken to heart when looking to buy: "A horse is no good without four good wheels."

Problems with the feet and legs will often result in the horse being unusable for your wife's equestrian activities. If less severe problems are found, a career of expensive, special shoeing and continuous veterinary costs to keep the horse sound enough to be ridden can still be the end result.

Last, but not least, make sure you buy a horse that your wife and family can handle. For first time horse owners, this is often a horse that is a little older and more experienced. My favorite quote from inexperienced horse buyers is, "we want to get a young horse that can grow up with our kids." I always want to respond: "So you don't like your children very much?" I never actually say that, but I do tell my clients that the chances of getting hurt with a very young horse is dramatically higher than with a more mature horse.

The bottom line is, always have a pre-purchase exam before you buy the beast because it will be a worthwhile investment.

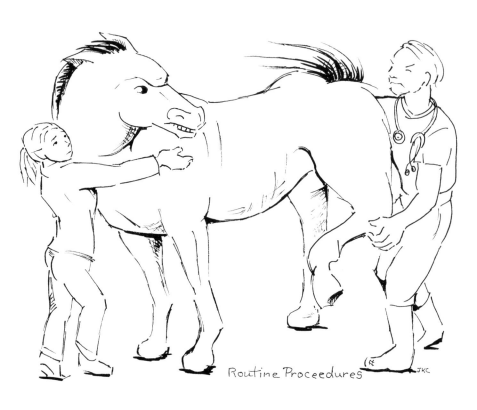

Routine Proceedures

Routine Procedures

"An ounce of prevention is worth a pound of cure."

Even though routine veterinary maintenance of the horse may not be your responsibility, as the horse husband, you need a brief overview to help you appear more informed at "horsey" cocktail parties.

All horses should receive vaccinations at least once a year, and possibly more often, depending on their situations. Equine vaccinations, much like those used for people, cause the recipient to be protected from the diseases they are most apt to get. When the animal is exposed to the disease it has been vaccinated against, its immune system kicks into high gear and attacks the offending pathogen. Spring vaccinations almost always include:

Tetanus – A bacterial infection that thrives in deep puncture wounds and causes muscle rigidity.

Encephalitis – A disease of the brain and spinal cord that is carried by mosquitoes.

Rhinopneumonitis and Influenza – Both are respiratory diseases that pass between horses like colds spread among kids in kindergarten.

Depending on the part of the country you live in, the horse may also need to be vaccinated against:

Potomac Horse Fever – A disease that causes diarrhea and leg swelling.

Strangles – A respiratory disease that leads to pus filled lymph nodes.

Rabies – A virus which causes neurological problems followed shortly by death. Rabies is contagious to humans.

Lymes Disease – A disease carried by certain types of ticks. Symptoms are similar to those in people, causing arthritis and fever.

West Nile Virus – Carried by mosquitoes, it causes staggering, lethargy and muscle tremors.

Equine Protozoal Myeloencephalitis – a parasite that gets into the spinal cord initially causing stumbling and may eventually lead to seizures.

Depending on what your veterinarian suggests, many horses will need to have at least some of these vaccinations repeated throughout the year.

De-worming, often referred to as "worming" should be done several times a year depending on your veterinarian's recommendation. This is another procedure that you will probably be recruited for. Some horses object to having a plastic tube filled with bad tasting paste shoved into their mouth. Trying to convince a 1000-pound animal that this is a good idea can get a little tricky.

Sheath cleaning is a procedure that may seem a little strange, but can be an important part of maintenance in male horses. Geldings and stallions can voluntarily retract their penis into their sheath which protects and covers it most of the time. In the normal horse, they will lower the penis out of the sheath to urinate. This is a good time to notice if his sheath needs to be cleaned. Within the sheath, lubricating oils are naturally secreted and can mix with dirt that is kicked up by the rear legs. Together, these substances form a waxy crud that will occasionally need cleaning.

Sheath cleaning helps to prevent infection and pain during urination. This procedure is most often performed with the horse under sedation to avoid being kicked by a very surprised male. Several good sheath-cleaning products are sold over the counter, but proceed with caution if you ever attempt this task.

Fresh out of veterinary school, an old gelding taught me a hard lesson about sheath cleaning and left me with a horse-shoe shaped bruise on my inner thigh that didn't go away for months. I hadn't given him enough sedative and paid the price. As they say, "Don't try this at home."

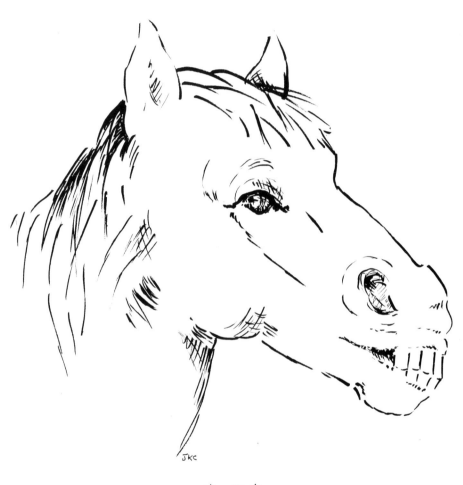

Dentistry

Dentistry

"Doc, he is dropping grain out of his mouth and has lost a lot of weight, you don't think it is his teeth do you?"

Oh yes, horses need dental work too. The most common procedure you may have heard of is called "teeth floating." No it doesn't involve a boat or raft. It basically means to file down the rough edges on the large chewing teeth in the back of the horse's mouth. These sharp "points" occur normally over time and can cause cuts in the cheeks and on the tongue if not occasionally filed off. The sores cause the horse not to chew its food properly, thus decreasing absorption, which may eventually lead to weight loss or even colic.

Sometimes more major dental procedures may need to be performed, such as molar tooth removal, but these problems usually occur in older horses. Removal of small ones, known as "wolf teeth," may need to be done more often because these little guys often interfere with the bit. A lot of head tossing or resistance to turning while riding may be a sign that these teeth need to be removed. Extraction of the "wolf teeth" can make the horse more comfortable and riding more enjoyable for your wife.

Most veterinarians will check the teeth when giving vaccinations and perform any necessary procedures. Equine dental work often requires at least some sedation to do a thorough job and keep every one as safe as possible. This is not a place to skimp to save money on your veterinarian's bill.

My most memorable equine dental experience came about as I was doing a routine float on a pony belonging to a five year old girl. The child had just recovered from some major surgery and the parents bought this old pony for her birthday. The pony was having a hard time keeping weight on, so I happily filed the sharp points off of its teeth just as I had done to hundreds of horses before.

I was almost done when the pony began to swirl its tongue, as if it was about to spit and then proceeded to spew three large teeth out on the ground in front of us! Of course the little girl immediately started to sob, sure that I had ruined her precious steed while the parents glared at me, waiting for answers. I gathered myself together and carefully explained that these teeth were rotten and needed to come out anyway. This was true, but I don't think they completely bought my answer. I now explain that this is a possibility before I start to float the teeth on an old horse.

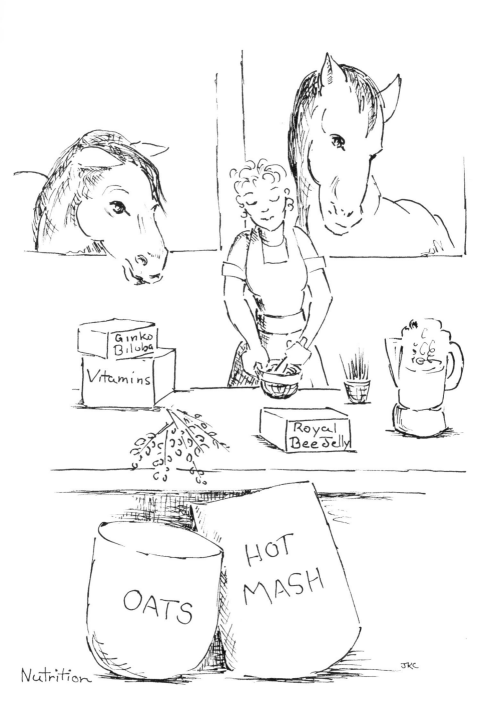

Nutrition

Nutrition

"The more I feed him, the more manure I have to scoop."

The best approach to nutrition is to consult with your veterinarian. Feeds, weeds, and nutritional problems vary widely from one region to another. However, there are a few general rules that apply to all horses which will help keep you in good graces with your wife and her horse.

First of all, never feed anything that is moldy or overly dusty. Feeds of this nature tend to make horses more prone to coughing and intestinal problems. Secondly, don't make abrupt changes in the amount of individual feeds. Whenever changing to a new or different type of feed, be sure to make these changes slowly. Mix a small portion of the new feed into the old to start with, and increase slowly.

When talking horse feed, more is definitely not always better. Try to stick to the same feeding schedule every day. If your wife feeds at 7 am and 6 pm, try to adhere to the same schedule if she can't be there. Last, but not least, I always recommend having a good mineral block available to the horse at all times. These very basic rules will keep you in good graces with your wife and the horse.

I once had a client's overzealous husband decide that a good way to get rid of some extra apples was to feed them to his wife's horses. His intentions were good, but his wife was away and the horses were not used to eating apples. After splitting an entire bag between them, he called me a couple of hours later;

both horses were having severe intestinal cramps and in need of immediate treatment. Paying me for my services was the easy part. Facing his wife's scorn was a much bigger price to pay.

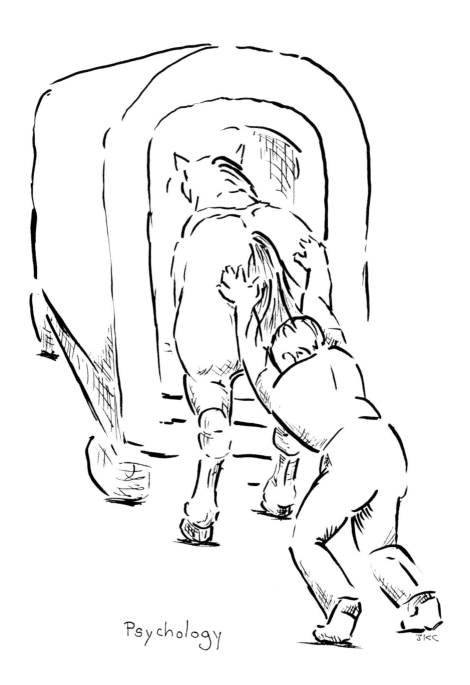

Psychology

Horse Psychology

"Doc, I don't think that horse has a brain in its head!"

In recent years, many new types of horse training techniques have surfaced. The older, "cowboy" ways have become passé, while new, more gentle techniques, using herd mentality, have become more popular. Most of these newer techniques use submission and dominance combined with the advantages of a round pen to tame the untamable.

I am not a horse trainer, but more of a "horse hollerer" than a "horse whisperer" so I will not delve much further into this subject. I would suggest, though, that the novice horse owner contact a good trainer to help improve the equine experience for all involved. You may want to carefully suggest this to your wife (even though she may not think she needs help), to improve her safety and maintain your happy home.

You may think that the mental health of your wife's horse is her problem, but trust me, on occasion, you will be asked to help her do something with the stubborn beast that may have required advanced preparation.

The most common situation that husbands are drawn into is the horse that won't get into the trailer. Horses always pick the worst possible time to pull this stunt, usually when your wife is in a big hurry to get to some form of equine event. I've had clients wrestle with their steed for hours and still not be able to get it into the trailer. They end up frustrated, and often with an injured horse and/or human.

Believe it or not, it does not help to cuss or threaten the animal with a trip to the dog food plant; these techniques have already been tried. The best plan of action is to get some horse psychology and training under your belt. The patience you show towards your wife's horse will win you praises and help keep the peace at home.

One of my favorite horsewoman phrases is, "My horse is afraid of men." I am a big, bearded guy, so there is no convincing a horse that I am a feminine creature. I cannot know if their fear comes from a previous abusive male owner, but without fail, these are most often the horses that want to kill me.

I did once have a horse that was truly afraid of me. He was tied in a line of horses waiting to be vaccinated. I vaccinated him just like the rest, but I noticed afterwards he started to act strangely. I immediately untied him and he proceeded to roll down the hill. Terrified, certain he had a major reaction to the vaccine, I scrambled down the hill after him. When I reached him I was prepared for the worst, but he started to get up. He shook it off and looked at me as if to say, "What is your problem?" then commenced eating grass.

The owner and I the put are heads together and realized that the horse had not taken a breath the whole time I had been working on him. He was so nervous about his vaccinations that he stopped breathing and fainted.

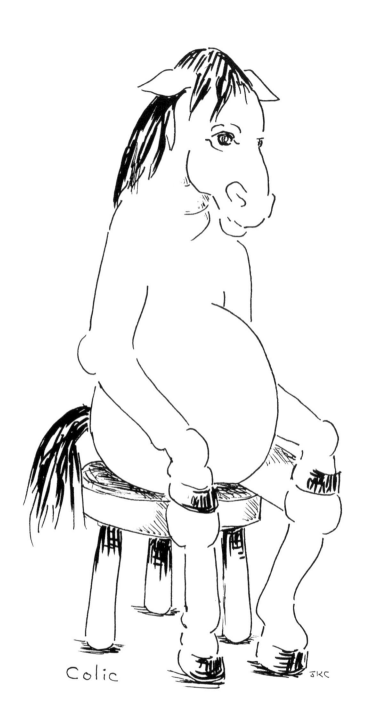

Colic

Colic

"I know it's midnight Doc, but my horse has been lying down and trying to roll all day so we thought this would be a good time to call."

The word colic often strikes fear into the hearts of the horse owner, but in many cases it is very curable when treated appropriately. Symptoms of colic include: restlessness, biting, looking at sides, lying down, trying to roll more frequently than usual, continuously striking the ground, and, in late stages, lethargy.

The general definition of colic is any condition that leads to abdominal pain. This may be caused by anything from constipation to a twisted intestine. The horse's intestinal tract is of relatively poor design. The equine digestive tract is a huge tube whose diameter changes in different sections producing the perfect environment for ingested food to get stuck in the more constricted regions. The huge volume of intestines is served by a relatively small amount of blood supply which does not allow distressed areas to receive the proper amount of blood flow.

Most colics can be relieved with painkillers, anti-inflammatories, and laxatives administered by your veterinarian. Laxatives are administered through a nasal-gastric tube into the stomach. Sedation is often required, since the patient is not thrilled about this procedure.

The most life threatening colics are the ones in which the intestines twist on themselves, or a section of intestine dies from loss of blood supply. Surgery is the best possible resolution for these conditions, but it may be very expensive and survival is not guaranteed.

My clients are always asking me, "Doc," what could I have done to have prevented this problem? In many cases, the answer is that we have no idea what was the underlying cause. At times, however, colic can be prevented. Dehydration, ingestion of too much grain, and severe parasite infections are often to blame. Additionally, horses that live in sandy environments are prone to ingest this sand if they eat directly off of the ground. When this occurs, the ingested sand can cause an intestinal blockage, creating a problem for your horse.

Equine practitioners tend to see more colicky horses when severe weather changes occur. Even though research has shown that weather does not effect the potential for colic, most equine practitioners will tell you otherwise.

For the anxious horse husband, what do you do when your wife is not there to get you and the horse through this? When a horse starts to exhibit colic signs, most veterinarians will tell you to start walking the animal. Keeping it up and moving will help gas and possible impactions to start moving, much in the same way that it feels good for us to take a walk after a big Thanksgiving meal. If you don't see any improvement in 15 to 20 minutes, or you can't even get the horse up and moving, it is time to call the vet. A word of advice, don't just watch the sick horse for hours before deciding to call your vet. We get pretty grumpy when called at midnight if we could have taken care of the problem during the day.

Another tidbit I should mention at this point: "Horse People" always want to give advice when a horse is suffering from colic. They seem to come out of the woodwork. While well-meaning, it is important to realize that some of them consider themselves experts after two weeks of horse ownership and may give you advice that varies from helpful to incredibly ignorant. Be smart, take all this advice "with a grain of salt," and don't delay in contacting the veterinarian.

Right after graduation from veterinary school, I was treating a colicky horse with an enterolith. An enterolith is a "stone-like" blockage in the intestinal tract that usually forms around a piece of metal or string that the animal ingested. My assistant and I had been up most of the night trying to keep the animal comfortable, without much luck. Suddenly, the exhausted animal stood up in the stall, raised its tail, and shot a grapefruit sized projectile across the room. My assistant awoke to the enterolith crashing into the cement wall of the building. The horse never missed a beat after that and went home with an ecstatic horse owner the next morning.

FEED

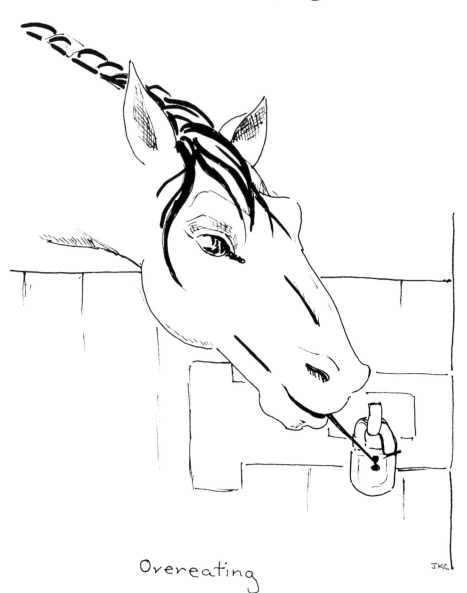

Overeating

JKC

Overeating

"Doc, there is no way he could have opened the latch to the feed room."

All too often, I get a call that a horse has broken into the feed storage area and as a result, is not feeling so well. Horses become great burglars when they can smell the feed behind the door. Their delicate lips can open the most sophisticated latch system. Some owners will even put two or three latches on at the same time and yet an occasional determined master thief will still get to the protected feed.

Horses seem to magically know when your wife is not home ensuring that you will be blamed for the whole fiasco. One of my clients had to resort to placing a "locked" padlock on the feed room door to deter a particularly slippery mare from gaining access. This was only after I had made three separate emergency trips to treat the same mare for overeating. Keep in mind, emergency trips are not free.

Ingesting too much hay is rarely a huge problem, but too much grain is almost always a recipe for disaster. It is often hard to determine how much was eaten when you discover what has occurred. Don't risk it. Alert your veterinarian as soon as you discover the break in. The accused will probably need to be treated with a combination of an injectable anti-inflammatory medication to help prevent laminitis and colic, along with a laxative to encourage the feed to move through quickly. The less feed that is absorbed, the less toxic the side effects. If you think the laxative can be simply offered to the horse and taken willingly with a glass of water, you are sadly mistaken. A plastic tube, several feet long, is stuck into the patient's nose and run down into its stomach, at which point, a voluminous amount of "ex-lax for horses" is literally pumped in. As you can imagine, a 1,000-lb. animal with teeth and hooves is not always easily persuaded to accept this procedure.

Treatment for this condition should be performed as soon as possible to keep permanent damage to a minimum. The "let's wait and see" approach is not a good choice here. You don't want to have to explain to your wife why you waited while the love of her life, (not you), needlessly died. No amount of veterinary bills is worth this potential end result.

The best prevention is to keep the grain and other feeds stored in a separate room or building with at least one good latch. Don't become one of those unsuspecting horse-owners whose critters get the best of them.

I actually had one client whose husband left the latch on the horse's stall unlatched three times in two weeks. Of course, I was called each time to treat the animal for overeating. By the time I arrived for the third treatment, the reluctant husband was already constructing a feed storage building as impenetrable as Fort Knox.

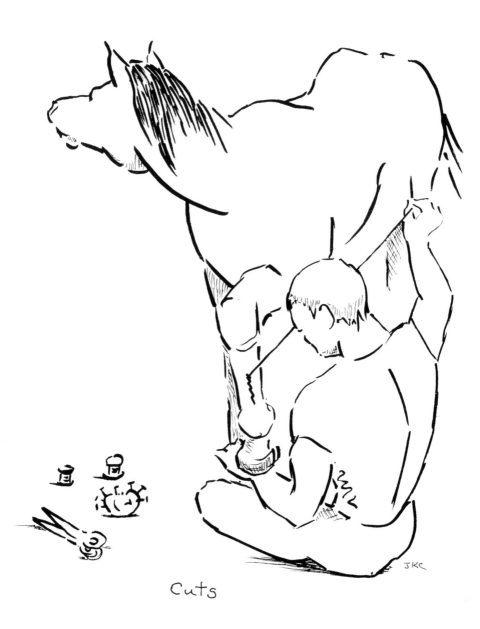

Cuts

Cuts and Lacerations

"Doc, he got cut real bad about a week ago, and we need you here right now."

Horses have an innate ability to find something to cut themselves on. It seems like they purposefully search out sharp objects in their living space to scrape against. The best prevention is for you and your wife to scour the stalls, paddocks, and pastures removing any sharp objects. The worst offender is barbed wire fencing. You will save yourself a lot of money and anguish if you replace it all with smooth wire immediately.

By removing as many dangerous objects as possible and always keeping an eye out for new ones that pop up, you can greatly reduce the chances of injury and make your life easier. Unfortunately, as most experienced horse owners will tell you, horses could be put in a padded stall and they would still find a way to hurt themselves.

The severity of cuts and lacerations vary greatly, but I will try to give you an idea of what is a "big deal." If a laceration has not penetrated the skin all the way through or is very small, it can probably wait a few hours, or until your wife returns home to be attended to. Exceptions are cuts or punctures over a joint, or wounds that bleed more than a slow ooze. If blood is squirting out of the wound for more than a couple of minutes, this quickly becomes an emergency. If you have any doubts about the severity of a laceration, consult your veterinarian and the two of you can decide what to do next.

It is a good plan to have some "first aid" bandage material on hand to control the bleeding until the vet can get to your horse. Wrap the area tightly until the bleeding stops or help arrives. This will make you a hero when your wife gets home. Try not to put any ointment or powder directly on the wound before the veterinarian arrives, because it will make it harder for he/she to clean up and suture the wound. Many larger cuts will have to be sutured closed for a couple weeks. Most lacerations need to be sutured within a few hours to increase the chances of proper healing. Sutures are usually removed in two or three weeks.

If your wife's horse is considered a show animal you may want to get help for even the slightest injury, otherwise the eventual scar and loss of ribbon may be held against you for a long time.

Another type of injury is referred to as a puncture wound. These are often caused by something long and sharp penetrating the skin and muscle then pulling back out again. Although this will need attention and cause a lot of swelling, it is not usually considered an emergency unless there is a lot of bleeding or if the wound is over a joint or tendon. If these wounds enter a joint they can cause severe infections and often result in permanent lameness if not treated promptly. I've had many clients who did not pay enough attention to these wounds, only to have severe problems later.

Always remember that if you don't feel comfortable dealing with a horse's injury, don't do anything that could damage you or the horse. Your wife may disagree, but you are not replaceable. A horse is a big animal that can do a lot of damage in a very short period of time. Too often, I have shown up to care for an injury, and both husband and wife are already limping from battle with the wounded beast.

One very busy Thanksgiving evening, I was called to look at a horse that ran a stick into its head while running through some timber. I assumed this would be an easy stop and that I could clean the wound and leave. Unfortunately, I had four more emergencies before this one, so I did not arrive until almost midnight. Much to my dismay I found the horse with the stick still in its head, looking much like a deformed unicorn. The "branch," as I referred to it, was approximately two inches wide and two-and one-half-feet long. I very carefully removed it, leaving a large hole in the animal's sinuses. By this late hour I was becoming a little "punchy." I leaned over, looked into the newly created cavern and shouted "hello, anybody in there." Much to my disappointment the owners did not see the humor in this move and a silence fell over the whole ranch. I quickly cleaned the wound, started the animal on some antibiotics, and sped away. I don't believe I was ever called back.

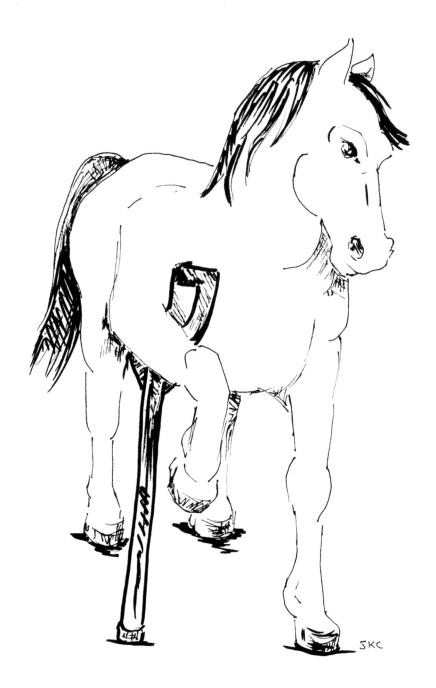

Lameness

Lameness

"He's been lame for about a week, so we rode him hard to loosen him up and now he is real sore!"

If you have been exposed to the "horse world" for any length of time, you have heard a collection of lameness nightmares. Horses can go lame for many reasons. Simply stepping on a rock or a nail can lead to a very sore foot. There are more causes of lameness than you could possibly imagine. For simplicity's sake, I will only give you a few examples.

Lameness varies as much in its severity as its causes. Essentially, if a horse is able to put some weight on the sore appendage, it is probably not an emergency and can be dealt with when your wife returns, or when you can get an appointment with your vet. The horse should be confined to a stall or small paddock, in the meantime, to prevent further injury. These types of lameness are most often caused by tendon and ligament injuries, bruises to the sole of the foot or minor trauma to the muscles of the leg. Minor lameness may also result from the loss of a shoe. In this situation, make an appointment with the farrier for a reset.

Minor lameness problems require you to restrict the animal's exercise until you talk to your wife or veterinarian. Most vets will recommend that you don't give the horse any pain medication until the underlying cause of the problem is found. Given incorrectly, pain relievers may temporarily mask the lameness and increase the chances of damage to the affected area. I tell you this to prevent you from having to sleep in the barn as punishment for improperly treating your wife's horse.

If the horse will not put any weight on the injured limb, you may have a more severe problem. The most common non-weight bearing injuries are foot abscesses and broken bones. Foot abscesses are best opened and drained by your veterinarian. They are usually quite treatable and rarely leave the horse with long-term problems. Injuries involving broken bones, however, are never as easy. This scenario often results in buying your wife a new horse. The take-home message here is, if the horse does not put any weight on an injured leg, call the veterinarian. Time may be of the essence!

I am often asked why broken legs in horses don't heal well. It is because the beast won't just lay down and elevate its leg for six weeks. Their sheer weight is just too much for a healing fracture to handle. Some fractures in smaller bones can heal with surgery or casting, but larger bones don't do as well.

A particular horse husband comes to mind when I think of lameness issues. His wife called me out to look at her barrel racing horse who was extremely lame the day before a big competition. I pulled in the driveway only to find the husband in the middle of re-roofing their house, a project that he was very proudly doing himself. Fortunately, this scene gave me a clue to the lameness diagnosis. I lifted up the sore foot and, as expected, a two inch roofing nail was protruding from the sole of the hoof. The husband's face dropped as I extracted the nail and his wife silently stared him down.

Although no words were spoken, he knew that his home improvement project would be blamed for losing the competition. Learn from his mistake and always be careful what ends up in the corral.

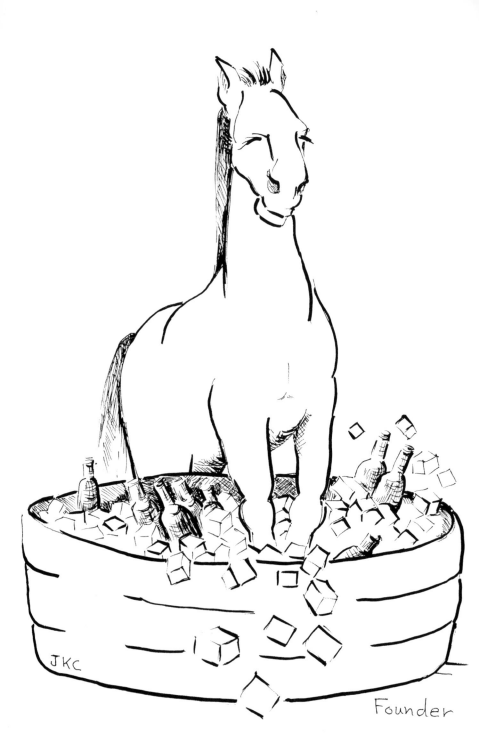

Founder

JKC

Laminitis

"Doc, my horse is real stiff on all four and doesn't want to move. Is it serious?"

Laminitis, or "founder," as it is called by most horse owners, can be caused by illness or injury, but is most often induced by overeating. Horses that are already overweight are more prone to founder. These factors lead to an inflammation in the hoof, which allows the bone inside the hoof, the coffin bone, to change positions. The result is pain in the animal's feet, often rendering it immobile. In most cases, the front feet are more affected. At times, when a horse is suffering from laminitis, they may lie down and be reluctant to get up. Laminitis can be fatal if the coffin bone moves too much. Ultimately, the coffin bone may come out of the bottom of the hoof rendering, the animal useless.

This situation can be recognized by stiffness in all four of the horse's feet. The horse may attempt to lean back in order to take as much weight as possible off the front feet and thus, relieve the pain. In some cases the hooves will also feel warm to the touch. Your veterinarian should be contacted immediately if you notice this condition.

While immediate attention is essential, be aware that treatment may become a long-term, expensive process, requiring frequent X-rays and special shoeing. Many horses recover quite well from laminitis.

I have some horses in my practice who "founder" every year in the spring. Their owners cannot resist turning them out onto the nice, lush, spring pastures. The horses quickly put on too much weight and develop laminitis. This is called "grass founder" by many and the end result is the same.

My own father has a small pony who cannot be turned out to pasture at all any more because it will eat itself to death. He now must keep it in a small dry lot, only feeding it a small amount of grass hay to prevent this problem from recurring.

I am always amazed when a client calls describing text book symptoms of a laminitis horse and swears that their horse is not overweight. Too often, upon arrival at their barn, I will find an obese horse, unwilling to move on very painful feet. Feeding a horse too much is almost as bad as not enough.

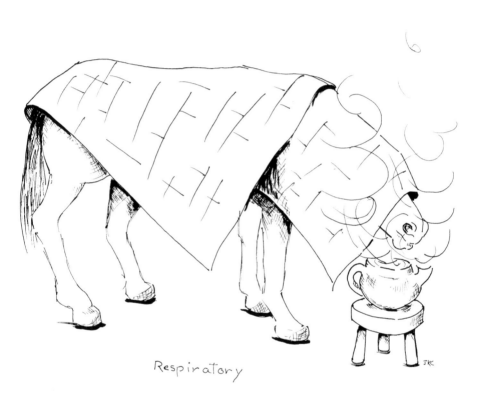

Respiratory

Respiratory Disease

"I thought he would get better on his own but now he has gotten worse and stopped eating. Can you save him Doc?"

Respiratory infections are quite common in horses and pass easily from one to another, similar to children in a kindergarten class. As in people, these infections are caused by viruses or bacteria in the lungs and respiratory tract, but do not normally transfer to people.

We routinely vaccinate for respiratory disease in horses, though they may contract different strains of the disease that are not covered by the vaccine. If your horse is coughing and discharging some opaque mucus, but is still eating normally, you probably don't have an emergency. It is when the animal loses its appetite and becomes depressed, or less active, that you are in trouble. The horse is likely to be developing a temperature and a veterinarian should be notified. You can take the temperature yourself, but he probably won't hold it under his tongue, so you'll need to go to the business end of the horse. I wouldn't recommend this unless you really know what you are doing.

Some horses may become so sick and weak that they start to lie down a lot. This is not to be confused with colic, where rolling is usually involved. These infections will often need to be treated by a veterinarian who can determine whether antibiotics or other medications will be required.

Another common respiratory problem in horses is very similar to emphysema in people. Horses usually don't smoke, but chronic exposure to dust and molds can have the same effect. This condition is often referred to as "Heaves." In horses, this usually shows up as a deep cough and commonly develops slowly over time. It often worsens during the drier times of the year. This condition warrants veterinary care, but is generally not considered an emergency.

I once was contacted by a couple whose horses had all developed a chronic cough. They were both medical doctors, so they had already tried to figure it out on their own before calling me.

When I pulled in to the barnyard, I found the horses munching their hay surrounded by a cloud of dust and molds. The hay was so old and moldy that I started to cough along with them.

Picking my words carefully, I began with, "You don't think it could be the dust do you?" Then the "light bulb" came on. While trying to hide their embarrassment, they sheepishly asked, "What should we do with the five tons of this hay we already have in the barn?"

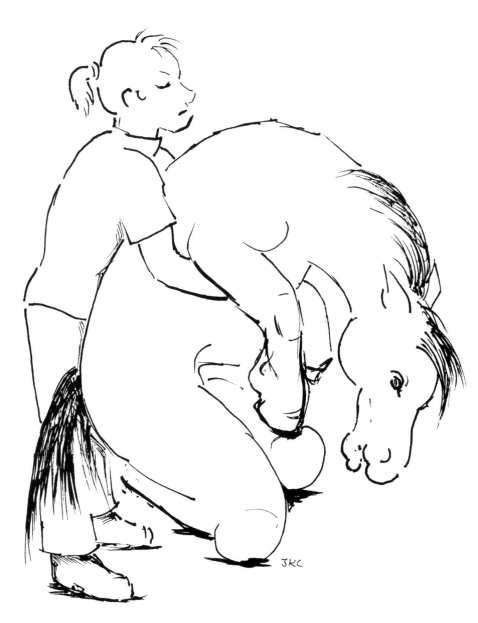

choke

Choke

"Hurry Doc, hay and grain are coming out of his nostrils!"

Choke is a condition that generally appears worse than it really is. The main symptom that you will notice is partially digested feed, mixed with saliva, flowing from both nostrils. This is caused by a blockage in the tube running from the mouth to the stomach (esophagus).

The most common culprit is pelleted feeds that are eaten too fast and not properly chewed. Horses with bad or missing teeth have a higher chance of having this occur. As a result of these conditions, the partially chewed feed gets stuck in the animal's esophagus and builds up into a hard plug. Everything the horse eats or drinks after the blockage is formed comes right back out the horse's nose.

This makes for a rather startling sight and you can understand why most owners panic. There is not much that you can do yourself to help the distressed beast, although sometimes rubbing the throat area will help to loosen things up. I wouldn't recommend trying the Heimlich maneuver or you may be the one needing a doctor.

Fortunately, your veterinarian can usually sedate the animal and pass a nasal-gastric tube to push the blockage into the stomach, clearing the esophagus. This procedure is not a particularly clean one, so don't wear your Sunday best. Usually by the time I have finished clearing a choke, everyone in a 20-feet radius is covered with slimy green, partially digested feed and horse saliva.

To help prevent choke in horses that eat too fast, some owners will put a couple of good-sized rocks in the grain bucket to force them to pick the feed out around the rocks, resulting in a more slowly-eaten meal. This, combined with good veterinary dental care, can decrease the chances of choke.

Occasionally, tumors or other abnormalities may be cause the blockage, but most chokes are relatively easy to treat. The bottom line is, choke is definitely a "call your veterinarian" situation.

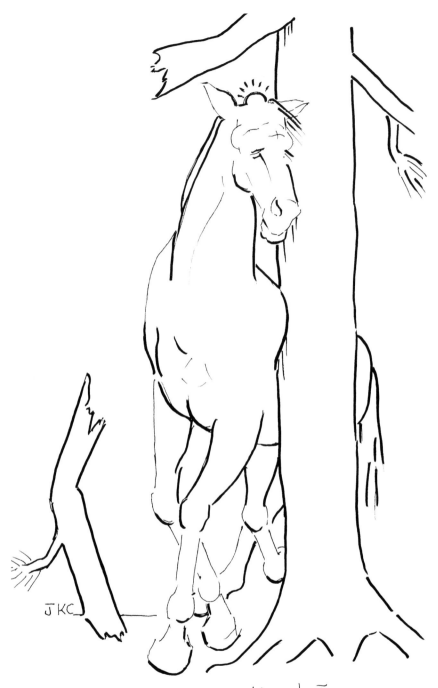

Head Injuries

Head Injuries

"He is such a big animal, I had no idea that such a small bump could affect him that much!"

I want to mention head injuries because they are probably the most dangerous to owners and caretakers. This condition is usually the result of a kick to the animal's head or contact with an immobile object, such as the top of the horse trailer. Sometimes it is hard to find the cut or abrasion, but underneath the skull, the brain may be swelling quickly as a result of the injury. This type of trauma is similar to head injuries people frequently receive in car accidents.

Outward signs of head injuries include staggering, blindness, and even seizures. A horse with any of these symptoms can be very dangerous to be around, so keep your distance if this occurs and contact your veterinarian immediately! A horse that is thrashing on the ground can pull you in with its legs and beat you up without even realizing what it is doing.

The phrase "my horse would never hurt me" does not apply in these situations. The horse will probably need steroids and other anti-inflammatories administered by your veterinarian. Prompt treatment is crucial for a good prognosis and to minimize self- inflicted damage to the horse.

Other conditions and diseases may cause these neurological symptoms, but most of these will come on more slowly, over time and not as dramatically.

I once went to check out a horse with minor abrasions to the head and face that appeared to be no big deal. When I examined the horse's wounds, I inadvertently raised the animal's head slightly and noticed his eyes start to roll upward. Shoving the owner over the half-door of the stall, I quickly followed, and we both looked back just in time to see the horse crashing over backwards right into the spot in which we had previously been standing.

We then realized the horse had a severe head injury and the mere raising of the head was enough to send him into a seizure. Needless to say, I am much more careful now when examining a horse with head wounds.

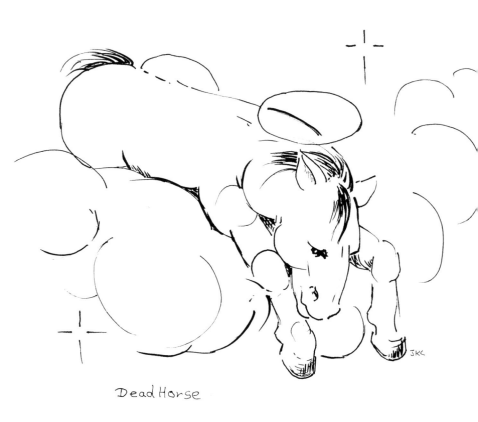

Dead Horse

Dead Horse

"I am sorry, we did every thing we could do."

Although this is a hard subject to discuss, realistically it happens to all horse owners eventually. It is often hard for people to understand that even though these animals are very large, they are relatively fragile. Horses, like other pets, become a part of one's family very quickly. Since your wife is spending the majority of time with the horse, she and the horse probably be the most closely bonded. If the horse dies, or has to be put down, it will definitely be the hardest on her.

Sometimes, when a horse is ill and shows no chance of recovery the veterinarian will euthanize the animal to put it out of its pain. This is usually done with an overdose of an anesthetic, a very painless and humane procedure.

The next problem you are faced with is how to dispose of this large body. In most areas, it is illegal or physically impossible to bury the corpse. The best course of action is to call an animal disposal company to come and pick it up. They will probably charge you a fee, but it will be worth every penny. If your wife is not at home when the horse expires, I would recommend that you cut off a handful of mane and tail hair as a souvenir for your wife to remember her horse by. Believe me, she will appreciate this later on.

It is also a good idea to know whether or not the horse is insured. If insured, a veterinarian postmortem exam is often required to determine the cause of death before the body is taken away.

Losing a horse can be very painful, but it is very important to keep things in perspective. An older veterinarian wisely reminded me once after I had euthanized a much-loved horse; "better in the barn than in the house." I try to keep that in mind whenever put in this situation.

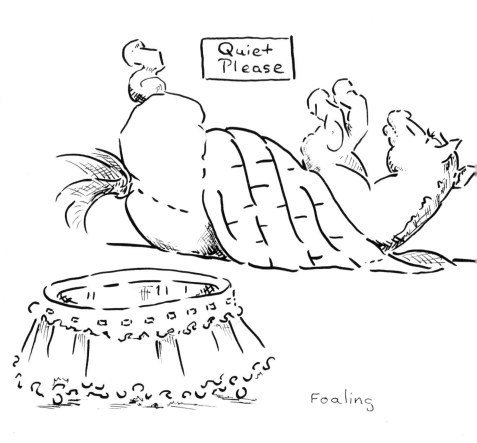

Foaling

Foaling

"Doc, I just ran into the house to grab some coffee and when I returned it was already born!"

If you are reading this section, you have probably embarked on a whole new adventure. Equine reproduction can be expensive and nerve-racking, so let me give you some basics to take the edge off.

Pregnancy can be diagnosed in mares at approximately 14 days by ultrasound and at 30 days by rectal palpation (yes, I said rectal). If pregnant, there will be special vaccinations and nutritional changes to be discussed with the veterinarian. Mares are pregnant for 11 months, although some can go longer or shorter.

During this time, your wife will become very worried about the upcoming birth and may even talk you into upgrading the mare's living area. One client of mine talked her husband into building three additions to their barn with an electrical upgrade before the foal was born. She then moved into the barn for two weeks, so as not too miss the big event.

Ideally, it would be best for your wife to be home for the birth. If she is away in Singapore, closing a business deal, let me offer some advice.

When the mare is close to giving birth, she will tend to be rather nervous and start getting up and down a lot. You may notice a waxy build-up or a milky discharge on her nipples. Eventually, a fluid-filled sack will emerge, followed by the foal itself. The front feet should come first, and then the nose. If the foal does not present this way, or is not making constant progress into the world, then a veterinarian should be consulted immediately.

Keep in mind that most foals are born during the night when no one is around or while you are in the house getting coffee. I have some owners that go as far as to set up video monitors in the stall to be sure they don't miss any of the action.

Assuming that the foal is born normally, make sure that the fetal membranes are pulled away from the foal's mouth and nose so they do not interfere with its ability to breathe. Let the mare clean off the rest because too much human intervention can make the mare nervous and increase the chances of injury to the foal or to you.

It is important to set the afterbirth aside for the veterinarian to inspect later. A manual inspection of the placenta will reveal whether or not the mare has fully passed the afterbirth. If she has not, your veterinarian will need to remove this, to prevent a uterine infection.

Within the first few hours, the foal should be up and trying to nurse. If this does not happen, another phone call to the veterinarian is warranted. It is most important the foal receive milk early, because the first milk contains many antibodies to help the foal fight off disease and infection. This early milk, also known as colostrum, contains lots of carbohydrates to help get the foal off to a good start.

Your wife should have left you an iodine dip for disinfecting the portion of the umbilical cord that is still attached to the foal and an enema for constipation (hopefully not yours). I can't count the number of times I have been called out for a foal that is not nursing, given it an enema, and had it shoot hard fecal pellets across the stall. The foal will then head right for the mare and start nursing, leaving the owner with my bill to pay.

Even if everything has gone well so far, you will still need to get a veterinarian to examine the foal within the first 24 hours to make sure everything is normal. This will help keep you out of trouble later if anything goes wrong.

Often owners are hoping for the foal to be a particular sex and are disappointed if they don't get what they wanted. Sometimes it is hard for the inexperienced eye to distinguish gender right after foaling.

Once I had a client decide that his wife's newborn foal was a stallion, which was exactly what she had been hoping for. It was destined to be a great breeding stud. He gleefully called her at work with the good news and proceeded to let all their horse friends know of the good tidings. A few hours later, I showed up to examine the new creature and announced that it was a very nice filly. After picking his jaw back up off the ground, he spent the afternoon reluctantly calling back those involved.

Glossary
(Helpful in Cocktail Conversation)

Bowed Tendon – Swollen tendon from some type of injury, usually on the back part of a leg.

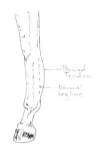

Brain – Very small when compared with other animals.

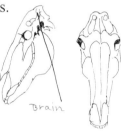

Brood Mare – Female horse used exclusively for raising foals.

Chestnuts – Cornified areas, one on the inside of all four legs.

Colt – Young male horse.

Cribber – Horse that chews on fences or posts.

Distemper – Old timers name for the disease "strangles."

Dressage – Specialized type of English riding.

English – European style of riding, done on an English saddle.

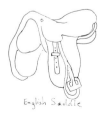

64

Farrier – Horse Shoer.

Filly – Young female horse.

Foal – Young horse of either sex.

Grade Horse – Any horse that is not registered with a specific breed association.

Gravel out – Pus from a hoof abscess that comes out at the top of the hoof.

Gelding – Castrated male horse.

Hand – Distance of four inches, used in measuring a horse's height.

Horse Poor – You, after your wife owns horses for some time.

Long in tooth – Horses teeth get longer with age.

Mare – adult female horse.

Navicular – Usually refers to a lameness problem caused by damage to the navicular bone in the foot.

Paint – A black/brown and white horse usually of quarter horse type.

Pinto – A black/brown and white horse of any breed besides Quarter Horse.

Proud Cut – A castrated male horse that still acts like a stallion and may still have a portion of its testicle left.

Quarter Crack – Crack on the side of the hoof that will cause lameness if deep enough .

Ringbone (High and low) – Arthritis in the first two joints of the leg, some will show a bump.

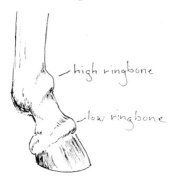

Spavin – Usually refers to arthritis in the hock joint.

Splint – Bump that appears on the inside of the front legs from stress in that area.

Stallion – Intact adult male horse.

Stocked up – Usually refers to swollen legs.

Stud – An intact adult male horse.

Three Day Event – English riding show that includes dressage, stadium jumping, and cross-country jumping.

Twitch – A tool that is placed on a horse's nose to keep his mind off whatever you are doing.

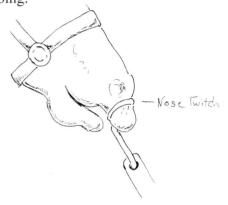

— Nose Twitch

Warmblood – Large horses, commonly used in English riding, and can usually be traced back to European draft horses.

Western – Type of riding that originated in the western United States, usually done on a western saddle(cowboys).

Windsucker – Horse that grabs fencing with front teeth and sucks in large amounts of air at the same time.

Epilogue

I hope this book has given you some insight into the world of horses and made you feel more comfortable. If you are left in charge of your wife's horse you should feel a little more at ease. Remember to always call the veterinarian if you feel a problem is out of your league. Your efforts will be appreciated for being overly cautious instead of neglectful. While horse ownership can be challenging and, at times, expensive, the rewards greatly outweigh the hardships. Enjoy the benefits of the good times horse ownership will give to you and your wife. If the boss offers you a raise, though, I recommend you take it!